111 Low Sodium Meal and Juice Recipes:

The Easy Way to Reduce Your Sodium Intake

By

Joe Correa CSN

COPYRIGHT

This publication is designed to provide accurate and authoritative information in regard to the subject matter covered. It is sold with the understanding that neither the author nor the publisher is engaged in rendering medical advice. If medical advice or assistance is needed, consult with a doctor. This book is considered a guide and should not be used in any way detrimental to your health. Consult with a physician before starting this nutritional plan to make sure it's right for you.

ACKNOWLEDGEMENTS

This book is dedicated to my friends and family that have had mild or serious illnesses so that you may find a solution and make the necessary changes in your life.

111 Low Sodium Meal and Juice Recipes:

The Easy Way to Reduce Your Sodium Intake

By

Joe Correa CSN

CONTENTS

ABOUT THE AUTHOR

After years of Research, I honestly believe in the positive effects that proper nutrition can have over the body and mind. My knowledge and experience has helped me live healthier throughout the years and which I have shared with family and friends. The more you know about eating and drinking healthier, the sooner you will want to change your life and eating habits.

Nutrition is a key part in the process of being healthy and living longer so get started today. The first step is the most important and the most significant.

INTRODUCTION

111 Low Sodium Meal and Juice Recipes: The Easy Way to Reduce Your Sodium Intake

By Joe Correa CSN

Most of the time people are concerned about the amounts of sugar in their diet, but large amounts of salt can also cause some serious health problems.

The main source of sodium in your everyday diet is salt. Unfortunately, most people are not aware of the amounts of salt they consume every day. Some statistics suggest that the average American eats five or even more teaspoons of salt every single day which is about 20 times more than what the body actually needs. This results in holding the excess fluid in the body which creates a significant burden on the heart followed by serious, life-threatening conditions.

Fortunately, this problem can easily be solved through a healthy diet and some small changes that will keep your health and well-being in check. Following a low-sodium diet means reducing the amounts of salt in your everyday meals which can easily be done while cooking. The actual problem lies in buying highly processed foods that often contain some ridiculously high amounts of salt. Make sure to check the nutrition labels of the foods you're buying when you go to the supermarket.

Adopting these healthy habits will reduce fluid accumulation in your body and ease the job of the kidneys which will result in significantly improved overall health.

Low sodium doesn't have to be low in taste! These recipes will give you an entirely new definition of flavor and will taste great.

This juice and meal recipe book is a wonderful collection of low-sodium juice recipes that I like to prepare for myself and I am sure you will enjoy and benefit from. They are full of flavor and nutrition.

111 LOW SODIUM MEAL AND JUICE RECIPES: THE EASY WAY TO REDUCE YOUR SODIUM INTAKE

JUICES

1.   Kale Grapefruit Juice

Ingredients:

1 cup of kale, chopped

1 whole grapefruit, peeled

2 cups of grapes

1 cup of watercress, chopped

½ cup of water

Preparation:

Combine kale and watercress in a colander and wash thoroughly. Chop it roughly using hands and set aside.

Wash the grapefruit and cut into chunks. Set aside.

Place the grapes in a colander and wash under cold running

water. Set aside.

Now, process grapes, kale, watercress, grapefruit, and grapes in a juicer. Transfer to serving glasses and stir in the water.

Refrigerate for 10 minutes before serving.

Nutritional information per serving: Kcal: 231, Protein: 6.7g, Carbs: 64g, Fats: 1.6g

2.   Cabbage Pumpkin Juice

Ingredients:

1 cup of purple cabbage

1 cup of pumpkin, seeded and peeled

1 large orange, peeled

1 large green apple, cored

1 tsp of ginger root

Preparation:

Wash the cabbage thoroughly and torn with hands. Set aside.

Peel the pumpkin and cut in half. Scoop out the seeds using a spoon. Cut one large wedge and peel it. Cut into small chunks and set aside.

Peel the orange and divide into wedges. Set aside.

Wash the apple and remove the core. Cut into bite-sized pieces and set aside.

Peel the ginger root and set aside.

Now, process pumpkin, orange, cabbage, apple, and ginger root in a juicer. Transfer to serving glasses and add few ice cubes.

Refrigerate for 10 minutes before serving.

Nutritional information per serving: Kcal: 228, Protein: 5.4g, Carbs: 69.3g, Fats: 1.5g

3. Strawberry Cranberry Juice

Ingredients:

1 cup of strawberries

1 cup of cranberries

1 small papaya, seeded and peeled

1 large lime, peeled

3 oz of coconut water

Preparation:

Place the strawberries and cranberries in a colander and wash under cold running water. Drain and set aside.

Peel the papaya and cut lengthwise in half. Scoop out the black seeds and flesh using a spoon. Cut into small chunks and set aside.

Peel the lime and cut lengthwise in half. Set aside.

Now, process strawberries, cranberries, papaya, and lime in a juicer. Transfer to serving glasses and stir in the coconut water.

Add some ice, or refrigerate for 10 minutes before serving.

Enjoy!

Nutritional information per serving: Kcal: 153, Protein: 2.6g, Carbs: 50.9g, Fats: 1.8g

4.   Radish Mint Juice

Ingredients:

1 medium-sized radish, sliced

1 tbsp of fresh mint, chopped

2 large pears, peeled and seeds removed

1 cup of blueberries, fresh

1 cup of cauliflower, chopped

¼ cup of coconut water, unsweetened

Preparation:

Wash the radish and trim off the green parts. Cut into small pieces and set aside.

Wash the pears and remove the core. Cut into bite-sized pieces and set aside.

Wash the blueberries under cold running water. Drain and set aside.

Trim off the outer leaves of cauliflower. Wash it and cut into small pieces. Reserve the rest in the refrigerator.

Now, process radish, mint, pears, blueberries, and cauliflower in a juicer.

Transfer to serving glasses and stir in the coconut water.

Add some ice and serve.

Nutritional information per serving: Kcal: 297, Protein: 4.9g, Carbs: 97g, Fats: 1.4g

5.   Brussels Sprout Leek Juice

Ingredients:

1 cup of Brussels sprouts, chopped

2 large leeks

1 medium-sized fennel bulb, chopped

½ tsp of fresh rosemary

Preparation:

Wash the Brussels sprouts and trim off the outer leaves. Cut into small pieces and set aside.

Wash the leeks and chop into small pieces. Set aside.

Wash the fennel bulb and trim off the wilted outer layers. Cut into small chunks and set aside.

Now, process Brussels sprouts, leeks, and fennel in a juicer. Transfer to serving glasses and sprinkle with finely chopped rosemary. Refrigerate for 10 minutes before serving.

Enjoy!

Nutritional information per serving: Kcal: 165, Protein: 8.5g, Carbs: 50.1g, Fats: 1.3g

6. Cranberry Spinach Juice

Ingredients:

1 cup of cranberries

1 cup of baby spinach, torn

1 cup of turnip greens, chopped

1 whole lemon, peeled

½ cup of pure coconut water

Preparation:

Place the cranberries in a colander and wash under cold running water. Drain and set aside.

Wash the baby spinach thoroughly and torn it with hands.

Wash the turnip greens and roughly chop it using hands. Set aside.

Peel the lemon and cut lengthwise. Set aside.

Now, process cranberries, baby spinach, turnip greens, and lemon in a juicer. Transfer to serving glasses and add pure coconut water.

Add some ice and serve immediately.

Nutritional information per serving: Kcal: 69, Protein: 4.3g, Carbs: 27.6g, Fats: 0.8g

7.   Radish Zucchini Juice

Ingredients:

1 small radish, trimmed

1 large zucchini, chopped

1 cup of red leaf lettuce, torn

1 medium-sized sweet potato, peeled

1 tsp of ginger, ground

Preparation:

Wash the radish and trim off the green ends. Chop into small pieces and set aside.

Peel the zucchini and cut it lengthwise in half. Scoop out the seeds and chop into chunks. Set aside.

Peel the sweet potato and place it in a pot of boiling water. Cook until fork-tender and remove from the heat. Drain well and set aside to cool. Chop into small pieces and set aside.

Wash the lettuce thoroughly and torn with hands. Set aside.

Peel the ginger root and set aside.

Now, process radish, zucchini, lettuce, sweet potato, and ginger in a juicer. Transfer to serving glasses and add some water to adjust the thickness, if needed.

Serve immediately.

Nutritional information per serving: Kcal: 67, Protein: 4.3g, Carbs: 18.6g, Fats: 0.8g

8.   Cauliflower Leek Juice

Ingredients:

1 cup of broccoli, chopped

1 small cauliflower head

1 large leek

1 cup of fresh kale, torn

1 large green apple, cored

2 oz of water

Preparation:

Trim off the outer leaves of a cauliflower. Cut into bite-sized pieces and set aside.

Wash the leek and chop into small pieces. Set aside.

Wash the broccoli and chop into small pieces. Set aside.

Wash the kale thoroughly under cold running water and torn with hands. Set aside.

Wash the apple and remove the core. Cut into bite-sized pieces and set aside.

Now, process cauliflower, leek, broccoli, kale, and apple in a juicer. Transfer to serving glasses and stir in the water.

Add some ice cubes and serve immediately.

Enjoy!

Nutritional information per serving: Kcal: 233, Protein: 12.7g, Carbs: 65.7g, Fats: 2.3g

9.   Banana Zucchini Juice

Ingredients:

1 large Granny Smith's apple, cored

1 large orange, wedged

1 large banana, sliced

1 medium-sized zucchini, sliced

2 oz of water

Preparation:

 Wash the apple and remove the core. Cut into bite-sized pieces and set aside.

Peel the orange and divide into wedges. Set aside.

Peel the banana and cut into small chunks. Set aside.

Peel the zucchini and cut in half. Scoop out the seeds and cut into small pieces. Set aside.

Now, process banana, zucchini, apple, and orange in a juicer. Transfer to serving glasses and refrigerate for 10 minutes before serving.

Enjoy!

Nutritional information per serving: Kcal: 296, Protein: 6.5g, Carbs: 86.8g, Fats: 1.7g

10.   Apple Cranberry Juice

Ingredients:

1 cup of strawberries, chopped

1 large Granny Smith's apple, cored

1 cup of cranberries

1 large carrot, sliced

1 whole lemon, peeled

1 large orange, peeled and wedged

Preparation:

Wash the apple and remove the core. Cut into bite-sized pieces and set aside.

Place the strawberries and cranberries in a colander and wash under cold running water. Drain and cut in half. Set aside.

Wash the carrot and cut into thick slices. Set aside.

Peel the lemon cut lengthwise in half. Set aside.

Peel the orange and divide into wedges. Set aside.

Now, process apple, cranberries, strawberries, carrots,

lemon, and orange in juicer. Transfer to serving glasses and stir in the water.

Add few ice cubes, or refrigerate for 10 minutes before serving.

Nutritional information per serving: Kcal: 268, Protein: 5.6g, Carbs: 89.1g, Fats: 1.6g

11.   Lime Cucumber Juice

Ingredients:

3 large beets, trimmed

1 large lime

1 large cucumber

2 celery stalk, chopped

1 small ginger root knob, 1-inch

2 oz of water

Preparation:

Peel the lime and cut lengthwise in half. Set aside.

Wash the cucumber and cut into thick slices. Set aside.

Wash the beets and trim off the green parts. cut into small pieces and set aside.

Wash the celery and chop into bite-sized pieces. Set aside.

Peel the ginger root knob and set aside.

Now, combine beets, lime, cucumber, celery, and ginger in a juicer and process until juiced. Transfer to serving glasses and stir in the water.

Refrigerate for 10 minutes before serving.

Nutritional information per serving: Kcal: 140, Protein: 6.7g, Carbs: 41.6g, Fats: 0.9g

12.   Sweet Orange Honey Juice

Ingredients:

1 large orange, peeled and wedged

1 cup of blackberries

1 large Golden Delicious apple, cored and chopped

1 cup of fresh mint, torn

1 tbsp honey

3 oz coconut water

Preparation:

Peel the orange and divide into wedges. Set aside.

Place the blackberries in a colander and wash under cold running water. Drain and set aside.

Wash the apple and remove the core. Cut into bite-sized pieces and set aside.

Place the mint in a bowl and add one cup of lukewarm water. Let it soak for 15 minutes.

Now, combine blackberries, orange, apple, and mint in a juicer and process until juiced.

Transfer to serving glasses and stir in the coconut water and honey. Add some ice and serve immediately.

Enjoy!

Nutritional information per serving: Kcal: 287, Protein: 5.3g, Carbs: 88.4g, Fats: 1.5g

13.   Cucumber Carrot Juice

Ingredients:

1 large cucumber, sliced

1 large carrot, sliced

1 cup of avocado, pitted and chopped

1 cup of pomegranate seeds

¼ tsp of nutmeg

3 oz of water

Preparation:

Wash the cucumber and carrot. Cut into thin slices and set aside.

Peel the avocado and cut in half. Remove the pit and cut into small chunks. Set aside.

Cut the top of the pomegranate fruit using a sharp knife. Slice down to each of the white membranes inside of the fruit. Pop the seeds into a bowl and set aside.

Now, combine cucumber, carrot, avocado, and pomegranate seeds in a juicer and process until juiced.

Transfer to serving glasses and stir in the water and

nutmeg. Add some ice and serve immediately.

Enjoy!

Nutritional information per serving: Kcal: 319, Protein: 7.1g, Carbs: 46.9g, Fats: 23.5g

14. Melon Banana Juice

Ingredients:

1 large Honeydew melon wedge, chopped

1 large banana

2 cups of green grapes

¼ tsp of cinnamon, ground

2 oz of water

Preparation:

Cut the honeydew melon lengthwise in half. Scoop out the seeds using a spoon. Cut one large wedge and peel it. Cut into small chunks and place in a bowl. Wrap the rest of the melon in a plastic foil and refrigerate.

Peel the banana and cut into small chunks. Set aside.

Combine green and red grapes in a colander and wash under cold running water. Drain and set aside.

Now, combine honeydew melon, banana, and grapes in a juicer.

Transfer to serving glasses and stir in the water. Add some ice before serving.

Enjoy!

Nutritional information per serving: Kcal: 374, Protein: 4.4g, Carbs: 105g, Fats: 1.7g

15.   Cranberry Apple Juice

Ingredients:

1 cup of cranberries

1 large green apple, cored and chopped

1 cup of strawberries, chopped

1 cup of fresh kale

1 large cucumber

Preparation:

Combine cranberries and strawberries in a colander and wash under cold running water. Drain and cut strawberries in half. Set aside.

Wash the apple and remove the core. Cut into bite-sized pieces and set aside.

Wash the kale thoroughly and drain. Torn with hands and set aside.

Wash the cucumber and cut into thick slices. Set aside.

Now, process cranberries, apple, strawberries, kale, and cucumber. Transfer to serving glasses.

Add some ice cubes before serving.

Enjoy!

Nutritional information per serving: Kcal: 229, Protein: 7.4g, Carbs: 72g, Fats: 1.9g

16. Carrot Grapefruit Juice

Ingredients:

1 large carrot, sliced

1 large grapefruit, chopped

1 cup of mango, chunked

1 large lemon, peeled and halved

1 small pear, cored and chopped

2 oz of water

Preparation:

Wash the carrot and cut into thick slices. Set aside.

Peel the grapefruit and divide into wedges. Set aside.

Wash the mango and cut into chunks. Fill the measuring cup and reserve the rest for some other juice. Set aside.

Peel the lemon and cut lengthwise in half. Set aside.

Wash the pear and remove the core. Cut into bite-sized pieces and set aside.

Now, process carrot, grapefruit, mango, lemon, and pear in a juicer.

Transfer to serving glasses and add stir in the water. Add some ice cubes or refrigerate for 5 minutes before serving.

Enjoy!

Nutritional information per serving: Kcal: 297, Protein: 5.7g, Carbs: 92.7g, Fats: 1.7g

17.   Collard Green Apple Juice

Ingredients:

1 cup of collard greens, torn

1 medium-sized apple, cored

1 medium-sized artichoke, chopped

1 cup of green peas

1 cup of carrots, sliced

2 oz of water

Preparation:

Wash the collard greens thoroughly and torn with hands. Set aside.

Wash the apple and cut in half. Remove the core and cut into bite-sized pieces. Set aside.

Using a sharp knife, trim off the outer layers of the artichoke. Wash it and cut into bite-sized pieces. Set aside.

Place the green peas in a colander and wash under cold running water. Drain and set aside.

Wash the carrots and slice into thin slices. Fill the measuring cup and reserve the rest for some other juice.

Set aside.

Now, process artichoke, green peas, collard greens, and carrots in a juicer. Transfer to serving glasses and refrigerate for 5 minutes before serving.

Nutritional information per serving: Kcal: 250, Protein: 16.2g, Carbs: 74.9g, Fats: 1.7g

18.   Apple Lettuce Juice

Ingredients:

1 large apple, cored

1 cup of red leaf lettuce, torn

1 cup of green beans, chopped

1 cup of fresh kale, torn

1 large lime, peeled

1 large red bell pepper, chopped

1 small ginger root knob, 1-inch

3 oz of water

Preparation:

Wash the apple and remove the core. Cut into bite-sized pieces and set aside.

Combine kale and red leaf lettuce in a colander and wash thoroughly under cold running water. Torn with hands and set aside.

Wash the green beans and chop into bite-sized pieces. Set aside.

Peel the lime and cut lengthwise in half. Set aside.

Wash the red bell pepper and cut in half. Remove the seeds and chop into small pieces. Set aside.

Peel the ginger root knob and set aside.

Now, process apple, red leaf lettuce, green beans, kale, lime, red bell pepper, and ginger root in a juicer.

Transfer to serving glasses and stir in the water. Add some ice and serve immediately.

Nutritional information per serving: Kcal: 194, Protein: 7.1g, Carbs: 52.9g, Fats: 1.7g

19.   Celery Carrot Juice

Ingredients:

3 large carrots, sliced

1 large cucumber, sliced

2 cups of celery, chopped

1 cup of sweet potatoes, cubed

1 small ginger root knob, 1-inch

Preparation:

Wash the carrots and cucumber.Cut into thick slices and set aside.

Wash the celery and cut into small pieces. Set aside.

Peel the sweet potato and cut into cubes. Fill the measuring cup and reserve the rest for some other juice. Set aside.

Peel the ginger knob and set aside.

Now, process carrots, cucumber, celery, potatoes, and ginger in a juicer.

Transfer to serving glasses and refrigerate for 5 minutes before serving.

Enjoy!

Nutritional information per serving: Kcal: 228, Protein: 7.6g, Carbs: 65.4g, Fats: 1.3g

20.   Squash Pomegranate Juice

Ingredients:

1 cup of pomegranate seeds

1 whole lemon, peeled

2 cups of butternut squash, chopped

1 large orange, peeled and wedged

1 cup of celery, chopped

2 oz of water

Preparation:

Cut the top of the pomegranate fruit using a sharp knife. Slice down to each of the white membranes inside of the fruit. Pop the seeds into a medium bowl.

Peel the lemon and orange. Divide orange into wedges and cut lemon lengthwise in half. Set aside.

Peel the butternut squash and remove the seeds using a spoon. Cut into small cubes and reserve the rest of the squash for some other recipe. Wrap in a plastic foil and refrigerate.

Wash the celery and chop into small pieces. Set aside.

Now, combine pomegranate seeds, lemon, butternut squash, orange, and celery in a juicer and process until juiced.

Transfer to serving glasses and stir in the water. Add few ice cubes and serve immediately.

Enjoy!

Nutritional information per serving: Kcal: 251, Protein: 7.3g, Carbs: 79g, Fats: 1.8g

21.　Cucumber Basil Juice

Ingredients:

1 large cucumber, sliced

1 cup of fresh basil, torn

3 cups of collard greens, torn

2 large carrots, sliced

1 medium-sized sweet potato, cubed

Preparation:

Wash the cucumber and carrots. Cut into thin slices and set aside.

Combine basil and collard greens in a colander. Wash under cold running water and drain. Torn with hands and set aside.

Peel the sweet potato and chop into cubes. Set aside.

Now, process cucumber, basil, collard greens, carrots, and sweet potato in a juicer. Transfer to serving glasses and refigerate for 10 minutes or add some ice and serve immediately.

Nutritional information per serving: Kcal: 201, Protein: 9.3g, Carbs: 57.3g, Fats: 1.5g

22.   Cauliflower Lime Juice

Ingredients:

1 cup of cauliflower, chopped

1 large lime, peeled

2 medium-sized tomatoes

1 large red bell pepper, chopped

3 oz of water

1 tsp of fresh rosemary, finely chopped

Preparation:

Trim off the outer leaves of cauliflower. Wash it and cut into small pieces. Reserve the rest in the refrigerator.

Peel the lime and cut lengthwise in half. Set aside.

Wash the tomatoes and place them in a bowl. Cut into quarters and reserve the juice while cutting. Set aside.

Wash the bell pepper and cut in half. Remove the seeds and chop into small slices. Set aside.

Now, combine cauliflower, lime, tomatoes, and red bell pepper in a juicer and process until juiced.

Transfer to serving glasses and stir in the reserved tomato juice and water. Sprinkle with fresh rosemary for some extra taste.

Refrigerate for 5 minutes before serving.

Enjoy!

Nutritional information per serving: Kcal: 98, Protein: 6g, Carbs: 28.5g, Fats: 1.3g

23.   Swiss Chard Cucumber Juice

Ingredients:

1 cup of Swiss chard, torn

1 cup of cucumber, sliced

2 cups of parsnips, chopped

1 large green bell pepper, chopped

1 ginger root knob, 1-inch

2 oz of water

Preparation:

Wash the Swiss chard thoroughly and torn with hands. Set aside.

Wash the cucumber and cut into thin slices. Fill the measuring cup and reserve the rest for later.

Peel the ginger and set aside.

Now, process Swiss chard, cucumber, parsnips, bell pepper, and ginger knob in a juicer.

Transfer to serving glasses and stir in the water.

Add some ice and serve immediately.

Enjoy!

Nutritional information per serving: Kcal: 219, Protein: 7.3g, Carbs: 68.8g, Fats: 1.5g

24.   Grapefruit Cucumber Juice

Ingredients:

1 large grapefruit, peeled and wedged

1 large cucumber, sliced

1 cup of papaya, chopped

1 small green apple, cored and chopped

2 oz of coconut water

Preparation:

Peel the grapefruit and divide into wedges. Set aside.

Wash the cucumber and cut into thick slices. Set aside.

Peel the papaya and cut lengthwise in half. Scoop out the black seeds and flesh using a spoon. Cut into small chunks and fill the measuring cup. Reserve the rest for some other juice. Set aside.

Wash the apple and remove the core. Cut into bite-sized pieces and set aside.

Now, process grapefruit, cucumber, papaya, and apple in a juicer. Transfer to serving glasses and stir in the coconut water.

Add few ice cubes and serve immediately.

Nutritional information per serving: Kcal: 246, Protein: 5.1g, Carbs: 72.4g, Fats: 1.3g

25.   Carrot Orange Juice

Ingredients:

1 large carrot, sliced

1 large orange, peeled and wedged

1 cup of cherries, halved and pitted

1 small apple, cored

1 whole lemon, peeled

2 oz of water

Preparation:

Wash the carrot and cut into thick slices. Set aside.

Peel the orange and lemon. Divide orange into wedges and cut lemon lengthwise in half. Set aside.

Wash the cherries thoroughly and cut into halves. Remove the pits and set aside.

Wash the apple and remove the core. Cut into bite-sized pieces and set aside.

Now, combine carrot, orange, lemon, cherries, and apple in a juicer and process until juiced. Transfer to serving glasses and add some ice before serving.

Enjoy!

Nutritional information per serving: Kcal: 253, Protein: 5.3g, Carbs: 78.2g, Fats: 1.1g

26.   Pumpkin Pineapple Juice

Ingredients:

1 cup of pineapple chunks

1 medium-sized zucchini

1 cup of pumpkin, chopped

1 cup of apricot, chopped

1 medium-sized apple, cored

2 oz of water

Preparation:

Cut the top of a pineapple and peel it using a sharp knife. Cut into small chunks. Reserve the rest of the pineapple in a refrigerator.

Peel the zucchini and cut in half. Scoop out the seeds and cut into cubes. Set aside. Peel the pumpkin and cut in half. Scoop out the seeds using a spoon. Cut one large wedge and peel it. Cut into small chunks and set aside. Reserve the rest for later.

Wash the apricots and cut in half. Remove the pits and cut into pieces. Fill the measuring cup and reserve the rest for some other juice. Set aside.

Wash the apple and remove the core. Cut into bite-sized pieces and set aside.

Now, process pineapple, zucchini, pumpkin, apricots, and apple in a juicer.

Transfer to serving glasses and stir in the water. Add some ice and serve immediately.

Nutritional information per serving: Kcal: 272, Protein: 7.2g, Carbs: 76.6g, Fats: 1.8g

27.   Mint Orange Juice

Ingredients:

1 cup of fresh mint, chopped

1 large orange, peeled

1 large green apple, cored

1 handful of fresh spinach, torn

3 oz of water

Preparation:

Combine mint and spinach in a colander and wash thoroughly under cold running water. Drain and torn with hands.

Peel the orange and divide into wedges. Set aside.

Wash the apple and remove the core. Cut into bite-sized pieces and set aside.

Now, combine apple, orange, mint, and spinach in a juicer and process until juiced. Transfer to serving glasses and then stir in the water.

Add some ice before serving and enjoy!

Nutritional information per serving: Kcal: 178, Protein: 4.4g, Carbs: 54.5g, Fats: 0.9g

28.   Cantaloupe Basil Juice

Ingredients:

1 cup of cantaloupe, chopped

1 cup of fresh basil, chopped

1 cup of cauliflower, chopped

1 cup of fresh kale, chopped

1 medium-sized cucumber, sliced

Preparation:

Cut the cantaloupe in half. Scoop out the seeds and flesh. Cut two wedges and peel them. Chop into chunks and set aside. Reserve the rest of the cantaloupe in a refrigerator.

Combine basil and kale in a colander under cold running water. Drain and roughly chop it.

Trim off the outer leaves of cauliflower. Wash it and cut into small pieces. Fill the measuring cup and reserve the rest in the refrigerator.

Wash the cucumber and cut into thick pieces. set aside.

Now, combine cantaloupe, basil, cauliflower, kale, and cucumber in a juicer and process until juiced. Transfer to serving glasses and add few ice cubes before serving.

Enjoy!

Nutritional information per serving: Kcal: 132, Protein: 8.9g, Carbs: 35.4g, Fats: 1.7g

29.   Lime Orange Juice

Ingredients:

1 cup of avocado, chopped

1 large lime, peeled

1 large orange, peeled

1 large cucumber, sliced

2 oz of water

Preparation:

Peel the lime and cut lengthwise in half. Set aside.

Peel the orange and divide into wedges. Set aside.

Peel the avocado and cut in half. Remove the pit and cut into small chunks. Fill the measuring cup and reserve the rest for some other juice.

Wash the cucumber and cut into thick slices. Set aside.

Now, combine lime, orange, avocado, and cucumber in a juicer and process until juiced. Transfer to serving glasses and stir in the water.

Add some ice and serve immediately.

Nutritional information per serving: Kcal: 132, Protein: 8.9g, Carbs: 35.4g, Fats: 1.7g

30. Kiwi Lemon Juice

Ingredients:

2 large kiwis, peeled

1 large lemon, peeled

1 cup of pineapple chunks

1 large carrot

1 large yellow apple, cored

1 tbsp of liquid honey

Preparation:

Peel the kiwis and lemon. Cut lengthwise in half and set aside.

Cut the top of a pineapple and peel it using a sharp knife. Cut into small chunks and fill the measuring cup. Reserve the rest of the pineapple in a refrigerator.

Wash the carrot and cut into thick slices. Set aside.

Wash the apple and remove the core. Cut into bite-sized pieces and set aside.

Now, process kiwis, lemon, pineapple, carrot, and apple in a juicer. Transfer to serving glasses and stir in the honey.

Optionally, add some vanilla extract for some extra taste.

Add some ice before serving.

Nutritional information per serving: Kcal: 132, Protein: 8.9g, Carbs: 35.4g, Fats: 1.7g

31. Spinach Orange Juice

Ingredients:

1 cup of spinach, torn

1 large orange, peeled

1 cup of butternut squash, cubed

1 large cucumber

1 ginger root slice, 1-inch

Preparation:

Wash the spinach thoroughly under cold running water. Drain and torn with hands. Set aside.

Peel the orange and divide into wedges. Set aside.

Peel the butternut squash and remove the seeds using a spoon. Cut into small cubes and reserve the rest of the squash for some other recipe. Wrap in a plastic foil and refrigerate.

Wash the cucumber and cut into thick slices. Set aside.

Peel the ginger root slice and set aside.

Now, combine spinach, orange, squash, cucumber, and ginger slice in a juicer and process until juiced.

Add some ice and water if necessary and serve immediately.

Enjoy!

Nutritional information per serving: Kcal: 209, Protein: 14.8g, Carbs: 61.6g, Fats: 2.1g

32.   Lime Orange Juice

Ingredients:

1 large lime, peeled

2 large oranges, peeled

2 large lemons, peeled

1 cup of fresh mint, torn

¼ tsp of pure peppermint extract

Preparation:

Peel the lime and lemons. Cut lengthwise in half and set aside.

Peel the orange and divide into wedges. Set aside.

Place the mint in a colander and wash thoroughly under cold running water. Drain and torn with hands. Set aside.

Now, combine lime, lemons, orange, and mint in a juicer and process until juiced. Transfer to a serving glass and stir in the peppermint extract.

Add some water if needed.

Refrigerate for 10 minutes before serving.

Nutritional information per serving: Kcal: 178, Protein: 5.8g, Carbs: 61.5g, Fats: 1.1g

33.   Lettuce Lemon Juice

Ingredients:

1 cup of red leaf lettuce, torn

1 large lemon, peeled

4 large carrots, sliced

1 large red apple, cored

Preparation:

Wash the lettuce thoroughly under cold running water. Torn with hands and set aside.

Peel the lemon and cut lengthwise in half. Set aside.

Wash the carrots and cut into thick slices. Set aside.

Wash the apple and remove the core. Cut into bite-sized pieces and set aside.

Now, process lettuce, lemon, carrots, and apple in a juicer. Transfer to serving glasses and add some ice before serving.

Enjoy!

Nutritional information per serving: Kcal: 231, Protein: 4.4g, Carbs: 70g, Fats: 1.4g

34.　Leek Broccoli Juice

Ingredients:

3 large leeks, chopped

1 cup of broccoli, chopped

3 cups of kale, chopped

1 large cucumber

1 small ginger root slice, 1-inch

Preparation:

Wash the leeks and cut into small pieces. Set aside.

Wash the broccoli and cut into bite-sized pieces. Fill the measuring cup and reserve the rest for some other juice.

Wash the kale thoroughly under cold running water using a colander. Drain and torn roughly chop it. Set aside.

Wash the cucumber and cut into thick slices. Set aside.

Peel the ginger root slice and set aside.

Now, process leeks, broccoli, kale, cucumber and ginger in a juicer.

Transfer to serving glasses and refrigerate for 10 minutes

before serving.

Nutritional information per serving: Kcal: 275, Protein: 17.2g, Carbs: 72.7g, Fats: 3.3g

35.   Grape Watermelon Juice

Ingredients:

1 cup of green grapes

1 cup of watermelon, seeded and chopped

1 cup of mango, chopped

1 large Fuji apple, cored

2 oz of water

Preparation:

Wash the green grapes using a colander and set aside.

Cut the watermelon lengthwise. For one cup, you will need about 1 large wedge. Peel and cut into chunks. Remove the seeds and set aside. Reserve the rest for some other juice.

Wash the mango and cut into chunks. Set aside.

Wash the apple and remove the core. Cut into bite-sized pieces and set aside.

Now, combine grapes, watermelon, mango, and apple in a juicer and process until juiced.

Transfer to serving glasses and stir in the water. Add few ice cubes or refrigerate before serving.

Enjoy!

Nutritional information per serving: Kcal: 288, Protein: 3.7g, Carbs: 80g, Fats: 1.5g

36. Pumpkin Pie Juice

Ingredients:

1 cup of pumpkin, chopped

1 cup of sweet potato, chopped

1 medium-sized carrot, sliced

1 medium-sized cucumber, sliced

1 medium-sized zucchini, chopped

¼ tsp of ginger, ground

Preparation:

Peel the pumpkin and cut in half. Scoop out the seeds using a spoon. Cut one large wedge and peel it. Cut into small chunks and fill the measuring cup. Reserve the rest for later.

Peel the sweet potato and cut into small chunks. Place in a potof boiling water and cook for 10 minutes. Remove from the heat and drain. Set aside to cool completely.

Wash the carrot and cut into thick slices. Set aside.

Peel the zucchini and cut in half. Scrape out the seeds using a spoon. Cut into bite-sized pieces and set aside.

Wash the cucumber and cut into thick slices. Set aside.

Now, combine pumpkin, cooked potato, carrot, cucumber, and zucchini in a juicer and process until juiced.

Transfer to serving glasses and stir in the ginger.

Add some ice and serve.

Nutritional information per serving: Kcal: 214, Protein: 8.3g, Carbs: 58.6g, Fats: 1.3g

37.   Guava Orange Juice

Ingredients:

1 large guava, chopped

1 large orange, peeled

1 large lime, peeled

1 medium-sized apple, cored

3 oz of water

Preparation:

Peel and wash the guava. Cut into small chunks and set aside.

Peel the orange and divide into wedges. Set aside.

Peel the lime and cut lengthwise in half. Set aside.

Wash the apple and remove the core. Cut into bite-sized pieces and set aside.

Now, combine guava, orange, lime, and apple in a juicer and process until juiced.

Transfer to a serving glass and stir in the water. Add some ice and serve immediately.

Nutritional information per serving: Kcal: 163, Protein: 3.5g, Carbs: 49.7g, Fats: 1g

38. Apple Orange Juice

Ingredients:

1 medium-sized Red Delicious apple, cored and chopped

1 large orange, peeled and wedged

2 large peaches, pitted and chopped

1 ginger root slice, peeled

1 tbsp of honey, raw

2 oz of water

Preparation:

Wash the apple and remove the core. Cut into bite-sized pieces and set aside.

Peel the orange and divide into wedges. Set aside.

Wash the peaches and cut in half. Remove the pits and cut into small pieces.

Peel the ginger root slice and set aside.

Now, process peaches, apple, orange, and ginger in a juicer. Transfer to serving glasses and stir in the honey and water.

Add a few ice cubes before serving and enjoy!

Nutritional information per serving: Kcal: 323, Protein: 5.6g, Carbs: 97.4g, Fats: 1.4g

MEALS

1.   Sweet Tropical Salad

Ingredients:

1 medium-sized mango, peeled, pitted, and cubed

3 large green apples, peeled and sliced

½ small pineapple, peeled and cubed

1 medium-sized cucumber, sliced

1 medium-sized orange, peeled and cut into wedges

For dressing:

1 tsp of fresh mint, finely chopped

2 tbsp of orange juice

1 tbsp of lemon juice

¼ tsp of paprika, ground

1 tsp of brown sugar

Preparation:

Place all dressing ingredients in a small mixing bowl. Stir

well to combine and refrigerate for 20 minutes.

Now, combine all other ingredients in a serving bowl. Mix well and pour over the dressing. Add one teaspoon of brown sugar for some extra taste.

Nutritional information per serving: Kcal: 165, Protein: 1.8g, Carbs: 24.5g, Fats: 0.8g

2.   Fresh Raspberry Overnight Oats

Ingredients:

1 cup of rolled oats

1 large peach, cut into small pieces

¼ cup of fresh raspberries

¼ cup of blackberries

¼ cup of almonds, finely chopped

2 tbsp of honey, raw

1 tsp of flaxseed

1 tsp of cinnamon, ground

Preparation:

Combine oats with one cup of water. Place in a deep pot and bring it to a boil over a medium heat. Cook for five minutes stirring constantly. Remove from the heat and chill for a while.

Place peach and berries in a serving bowl. Add oatmeal and stir to combine.

Meanwhile, combine honey with flaxseed and almonds in a small bowl. Pour the mixture over oatmeal and sprinkle with some cinnamon.

Refrigerate overnight.

Nutritional information per serving: Kcal: 166, Protein: 4.1g, Carbs: 41.4g, Fats: 2.3g

3. Tomatoes 'n Cheese Mini- Skewers

Ingredients:

4 oz of cherry tomatoes, halved

5 oz of Mozzarella cheese balls

1 cup fresh basil leaves, whole

3 tbsp of extra virgin olive oil

¼ tsp of black pepper, ground

½ tsp of balsamic vinegar

Skewers

Preparation:

String tomato, one leaf of basil, and one cheese ball onto a toothpick. Repeat the process until you run out of ingredients. Transfer the skewers to the serving plate.

Season with pepper, olive oil, and balsamic vinegar.

Serve immediately.

Nutritional information per serving: Kcal: 172, Protein: 8.2g, Carbs: 11.6g, Fats: 21.4g

4.   Spicy Veal and Watermelon Salad

Ingredients:

5 oz of veal steak, thinly sliced

½ small watermelon, peeled and cubed

1 medium-sized red onion, sliced

1 tbsp of fresh mint

¼ tsp of black pepper, ground

For dressing:

2 tbsp of olive oil

1 tsp of red pepper, crushed

3 tbsp of lemon juice

1 tsp of fresh cilantro

1 tsp of honey

Preparation:

Preheat the olive oil in a large frying pan over a medium-high temperature. Add the onion and stir-fry for about 2 minutes. Now add the veal slices and sprinkle with ground pepper to taste. Grill until meat is medium-rare or until charcoal edges.

Combine dressing ingredients in a mixing bowl. Stir well with a whisk and set aside.

Transfer the meat and onion on a serving plate and arrange watermelon and mint over it.

Drizzle the salad with dressing and serve.

Nutritional information per serving: Kcal: 180, Protein: 15.2g, Carbs: 14.3g, Fats: 9.3g

5.   Sesame Seed Chicken

Ingredients:

1 lb of chicken breasts, skinless and boneless, thinly sliced

2 large eggs

4 oz of sesame seeds

4 oz of breadcrumbs

1 tsp of Cayenne pepper, ground

1 tbsp of fresh parsley, finely chopped

1 tbsp of olive oil

Preparation:

Whisk the eggs, sesame seeds and breadcrumbs in a mixing bowl. Stir well and set aside.

Preheat the oil in a large frying pan over a medium-high temperature. Add chicken slices and cook for about 10 minutes from both sides. Now, pour over egg mixture and reduce temperature to low. Cook for 4-5 minutes more and remove from the heat. Transfer to the serving plate and sprinkle with fresh parsley.

Serve with some fresh vegetables.

Nutritional information per serving: Kcal: 250, Protein: 8.6g, Carbs: 28.7g, Fats: 10.3g

6.   Vanilla Strawberry Smoothie

Ingredients:

1 cup of skim milk

1 tsp of vanilla extract

½ cup of strawberries, halved

1 tbsp of almonds, finely chopped

1 tbsp of sugar

2 tsp of honey

Preparation:

Combine all ingredients in a blender. Blend until smooth. Transfer to a large glass. Refrigerate at least one hour before using.

Serve with fresh fruits by your choice.

Enjoy!

Nutritional information per serving: Kcal: 270, Protein: 4.5g, Carbs: 78.3g, Fats: 0.1g

7.   Grilled Veal and Mushroom Risotto

Ingredients:

1 lb of veal, skinless and boneless

3 large onions, chopped

1 cup of button mushrooms, halved

1 cup of white rice

1 tbsp of parsley, finely chopped

1 tsp of black pepper, ground

3 medium-sized tomatoes, chopped

2 garlic cloves, finely chopped

1 tsp of red pepper, ground

2 tbsp of olive oil

Preparation:

Preheat one tablespoon of oil in a large skillet over a medium temperature. Add the onions and str-fry for about 4-5 minutes or until translucent. Add the mushrooms and stir well. Cook for 10 minutes and then add rice. Stir once again and cook for 2 more minutes. Now add water until it covers all ingredients. Cover with a lid, reduce temperature to low and cook for 15 minutes. Remove from the heat and stir in parsley. Set the risotto aside.

Preheat one tablespoon of oil in a large skillet over a medium-high temperature.Using your hands, rub in the pepper and red pepper to the veal chops. Place the meat in the skillet and cook for about 10 minutes from both sides, or until crisp.

Meanwhile, place the tomatoes in the food processor. Blend until smooth and pour the mixture into the skillet.

Add one cup of water, cover with a lid, and reduce the heat to low. Cook for 25-30 minutes and remove from the heat.

Serve meat and risotto with some fresh salad.

Nutritional information per serving: Kcal: 504, Protein: 32.3g, Carbs: 48.3g, Fats: 21.2g

8.   Hot Mexican Salad

Ingredients:

1 lb of red bell peppers, halved

3 tbsp of olive oil

3 large onions, chopped

4 medium-sized tomatoes, chopped

1 tsp of fresh coriander, finely chopped

1 small chili pepper, finely chopped

2 tbsp of fresh spring onions, chopped

2 tbsp of lime juice

¼ tsp of black pepper, ground

½ tbsp of vegetable vinegar

Preparation:

Preheat the oven to 400°F. Grease the baking sheet with olive oil and place peppers. Bake for 10 minutes. Remove from the oven and set aside to cool. Remove the seeds and peel.

Combine peppers and onion in a large bowl. Mix vinegar,

oil and ¼ cup of water. Stir well and marinate for 2 hours.

Now, combine tomatoes, pepper, chili, coriander and spring onions into another bowl.

Transfer the peppers and onions to the serving plate. Top with tomatoes and spices mixture.

You can pour over the marinade juice for extra flavor.

Nutritional information per serving: Kcal: 165, Protein: 4.1g, Carbs: 19.5g, Fats: 9.7g

9.　Red Pepper Baked Potatoes

Ingredients:

1 lb of medium-sized potatoes, peeled and halved

4 tbsp of olive oil

2 large tomatoes, chopped

1 tsp of red pepper, ground

1 tsp of fresh parsley, finely chopped

1 tsp of balsamic vinegar

Preparation:

Preheat the oven to 400°F.

Grease large baking sheet with 1 tbsp of olive oil. Place the potatoes and season with red pepper. Bake for 15 minutes, or until crisp. Remove from the heat and set aside to cool.

Meanwhile, transfer tomatoes, parsley, oil, and vinegar to a food processor. Blend until smooth and set the sauce aside.

Transfer potatoes to the serving plate. Top with sauce and serve.

Nutritional information per serving: Kcal: 300, Protein: 6.1g, Carbs: 58.4g, Fats: 9.3g

10.   Delicious Beef Pot

Ingredients:

1 lb of lean beef, chopped into bite-sized pieces

2 medium-sized onions, chopped

1 bell pepper, seeds removed and chopped

3 large potatoes, peeled and chopped

1 cup of button mushrooms, halved

2 tbsp of vegetable oil

½ tsp of black pepper, ground

1 tsp of Cayenne pepper, ground

1 tsp of all-purpose flour

1 tsp of parsley

½ tsp of sugar

Preparation:

Place meat into a large pot or a pressure cooker. Pour some water until covers the meat. Cover with a lid and cook for 15 minutes on a medium temperature.

Remove from the heat and set aside without lid.

Meanwhile, preheat the oil in a large frying skillet over a medium temperature. Add mushrooms, potatoes, and sprinkle with sugar. Cook for 5 minutes and transfer all to the pot. Now, add all remaining ingredients and give it a final stir.

Cook for 30 minutes on a medium temperature. Remove from the heat and cool.

Serve.

Nutritional information per serving: Kcal: 209, Protein: 17.2g, Carbs: 25.8g, Fats: 7.3g

11.   Grilled Mussel Salad

Ingredients:

2 lbs of fresh mussels, debearded

1 large onion, peeled and finely chopped

3 cloves of garlic, crushed

4 tbsp of olive oil

¼ cup of fresh parsley, finely chopped

1 tbsp of rosemary, finely chopped

1 cup of lamb's lettuce

½ cup of arugula leaves

1 large cherry tomato, for decoration

Preparation:

Rinse and drain the mussels. Set aside.

Heat up the olive oil over medium-high temperature. Peel and finely chop the onion. Reduce the heat to medium temperature and add the chopped onion. Stir-fry for several minutes, until crisp-tender. Now add the mussels and finely chopped parsley. Cook for about 20 minutes, shaking the skillet regularly. When all the water has evaporated, add garlic, chopped rosemary and mix well again.

In a large bowl, combine the mussels with lamb's lettuce. Add the remaining oil, and decorate with one cherry tomato.

Serve immediately.

Nutritional information per serving: Kcal: 192, Protein: 18.2g, Carbs: 8.9g, Fats: 42.2g

12. Cauliflower Soup with Garlic

Ingredients:

1 large head cauliflower, cut into bite-sized pieces

1 tbsp vegetable oil

1 garlic clove, crushed

1 leek, chopped

1 tbsp of butter

4 fl oz vegetable broth, unsalted

½ cup of fresh Mozzarela cheese, unsalted

Preparation:

Place cauliflower and cheese into the food processor. Blend for 30 seconds and set aside.

Heat the oil in a large pot over a medium-high temperature. Add butter, garlic and leek and saute for 2-3 minutes.

Transfer the caliuflower and cheese mixture to the pot and add the vegetable broth. Cover, reduce the heat to minimum and cook for 25 minutes.

Serve warm.

Nutritional information per serving: Kcal: 132, Protein: 9.3g, Carbs: 21.4g, Fats: 7.9g

13.   Watercress Salad with Parsley Root

Ingredients:

7oz parsley root, sliced

3.5oz watercress, torn

1oz Mozzarella cheese, unsalted

1 tbsp of sunflower seeds

1 tbsp of apple cider vinegar

2 tbsp of extra virgin olive oil

1 garlic clove, crushed

Preparation:

Place the sliced parsley root in a pot. Add enough water to cover and cook until soft. This should take about 45 minutes.

You can speed up the process and reduce the cooking time if you place the parsley root in a pressure cooker. Set for 10 minutes on high. Remove from the heat.

Heat up one tablespoon of olive oil and stir-fry the root for 3-4 minutes. Set aside.

Wash watercress and roughly chop. Place in a large bowl.

Add cooked parsley root and mix well.

In a small bowl, combine the olive oil with apple cider, and garlic. Stir well and drizzle over salad.

Serve with sunflower seeds and cheese.

Nutritional information per serving: Kcal: 74, Protein: 3.8g, Carbs: 16.7g, Fats: 1.5g

14.   Simple Tomato Soup

Ingredients:

4 large tomatoes, peeled and roughly chopped

1 tbsp of celery, finely chopped

1 medium-sized onion, diced

1 tbsp of fresh basil, finely chopped

2 tbsp of extra virgin olive oil

½ tsp of black pepper, ground

½ tsp of sugar

Fresh water

Preparation:

Heat up the olive oil in a non-stick frying pan over a medium-high temperature. Add the onions, celery, and fresh basil. Sprinkle with some pepper and stir-fry for about 10 minutes, until caramelized.

Add the tomato and about ¼ cup of water. Reduce the heat to minimum and cook for about 15 minutes, until softened. Now add about 1 cup of water and 1 teaspoon of sugar and bring it to a boil. Remove from the heat and serve with fresh parsley.

Nutrition information per serving: Kcal: 89, Protein: 0.7g, Carbs: 4.9g, Fats: 7g

15.   Beef Soup with Veggies

Ingredients:

1 pound chicken breast, boneless and skinless, chopped into bite-sized pieces

1 onion, peeled and finely chopped

1 carrot, sliced

2 tbsp of almond flour

1 tsp of cayenne pepper

2 egg yolks

3 tbsp of freshly squeezed lemon juice

3 tbsp of extra-virgin olive oil

4 cups of vegetable broth

Preparation:

Heat the oil in pressure cooker, over medium-high heat. Stir fry the onion until translucent.

Now add sliced carrot, cayenne pepper and continue to cook for 3 more minutes.

Add other ingredients, pour broth and mix well.

Securely lock the cooker and set the heat to high for 20 minutes.

Nutrition information per serving: Kcal: 140, Protein: 17g, Carbs: 13g, Fats: 9g

16.   Hokkaido Pumpkin Salad

Ingredients:

½ small Hokkaido pumpkin, cut in cubes

3 oz of salmon, thin sliced

½ cup of baby spinach, finely chopped

½ cup of walnuts

1 tbsp of olive oil

1 tbsp of lemon juice

¼ tsp of ground pepper

Preparation:

First, preheat the oven to 520°F.

Now, peel the pumpkin and cut into bite-sized cubes. Line some baking paper over a baking sheet. I like to grease my baking paper with some olive oil, but this is optional. Put the pumpkin cubes in it, and add some salt and pepper. Bake for about 10 minutes, or until charcoal edges.

Preheat a non-stick frying pan over a medium-high temperature. Add smoked salmon slices and grill until nice and crispy on both sides. Remove from the pan and set aside.

Spread the baby spinach over a serving plate. Make a layer with chopped pumpkin and smoked salmon. Top with walnuts and sprinkle with lemon juice, olive oil, and pepper to taste. Serve immediately!

Nutritional information per serving: Kcal: 306, Protein: 13.7g, Carbs: 6.9g, Fats: 25.2g

17.   Chicken in Mushroom Sauce

Ingredients:

1 pound of chicken meat, skinless

2 tbsp of all-purpose flour

1 cup of button mushrooms

1 cup of green beans, cooked

¼ cup of chicken broth

½ tsp of sea salt

¼ tsp of black pepper

4 tbsp of olive oil

Preparation:

Wash and pat dry the chicken meat. In a large bowl, combine all-purpose flour with salt and pepper. Coat the chicken with the flour and set aside. Heat up the olive oil over a medium temperature and fry chicken meat for about 5 minutes on each side. Remove from the saucepan and transfer to a plate. In the same saucepan add chicken broth, green beans, and button mushrooms. Bring it to a boil and cook for 2-3 minutes. Return the chicken and cook for another 20 minutes, stirring occasionally, until the water evaporates. Serve warm.

Nutritional information per serving: Kcal: 331, Protein: 41.3g, Carbs: 18.5g, Fats: 10.4g

18.   Winter Salad

Ingredients:

2 large pears, peeled and cut into wedges

2 large oranges, peeled and cut into wedges

¼ cup of dried figs, chopped

¼ cup of dried apricots, chopped

¼ tsp of cinnamon, ground

½ tsp of walnuts, ground and unsalted

1 cup of lime juice

Preparation:

Combine all fruits in a large serving bowl. Mix all well and set side.

Meanwhile, combine cinammon and walnuts in a mixing bowl. Add lime juice and spoon well. Pour over the dressing over fruit and refrigerate for about 30 minutes.

Serve.

Nutritional information per serving: Kcal: 201, Protein: 2.2g, Carbs: 71.3g, Fats: 0.5g

19. Eggplant Soup

Ingredients:

3 small eggplants, peeled and cut into bite-sized pieces

1 medium-sized red onion, finely chopped

2 medium sized tomatoes, peeled and chopped

1 tbsp of sour cream

3 tbsp of olive oil

½ tsp of black pepper, ground

¼ tsp of chili pepper, ground

Preparation:

Put eggplant cubes in a large bowl, and add some salt. Set aside for about 15 minutes (salt will take out the bitterness). Wash the eggplants and dry with kitchen paper.

Heat up some olive oil in a frying pan over medium-high temperature. Add finely chopped onion and stir fry until translucent. Add eggplant chunks and stir fry for few minutes.

Add tomatoes in a frying pan and stir well. Cook for about

3-4 minutes more, remove from the heat and cool for a while. Transfer to the food processor and blend until smooth.

Take a large deep pot and transfer the mixture from the food processor. Add 2 fl oz of water, pepper, chili, and cover with a lid. Cook for about minutes.

Serve warm.

Nutritional information per serving: Kcal: 125, Protein: 5.6g, Carbs: 17.4g, Fats: 19.7g

20.   Veggie Pockets

Ingredients:

6 oz of cauliflower, chopped

2 bell peppers, seeds removed, cut into strips

2 small carrots, sliced

1 small zucchini, peeled and chopped

6 oz of brussel sprouts, halved

4 garlic cloves, finely chopped

1 tsp of basil, finely chopped

½ tsp of black pepper, ground

2 tbsp of olive oil

Preparation:

Preheat the oven to 400°F.

Combine all ingredients in a large mixing bowl. Stir well to combine. Sprinkle with olive oil.

Divide the mixtures into 4 equal sizes onto aluminum foil. Bring up 2 sides of foil so edges meet. Seal edges, allowing space for heat circulation.

Transfer wraps to a large baking sheet. Bake for about 50 minutes. Remove from the oven and set aside to cool.

Enjoy!

Nutritional information per serving: Kcal: 74, Protein: 5.6g, Carbs: 13.8g, Fats: 12.1g

21. Meatballs with Capers Gravy

Ingredients:

1 lb of ground beef

1 medium-sized onion, chopped

3 tbsp of olive oil

2 egg yolks

1 tsp of fresh bay leaf, finely chopped

2 oz of capers

½ tsp of black pepper

2 tbsp of lemon juice

Fresh water

Preparation:

Mix the ground beef with the eggs, black pepper, olive oil, and onion so that they all combine nicely. Roll the ground beef into small balls with your hand and place them on a medium heat pan. Cook them for 3-10 minutes or until you see there is no red in the interior of the balls.

In a separate pot, combine 2 cups of water, lemon juice, capers, and bay leaf. Bring it to a boil and carefully add meatballs with a spoon. Cook for 15 minutes and transfer the meatballs to the serving plate. Reserve the water.

Nutritional information per serving: Kcal: 158, Protein: 14.7g, Carbs: 13.6g, Fats: 9.1g

22.   Italian Wild Asparagus Salad

Ingredients:

8 oz of fresh asparagus, whole

3 tbsp of tuna, oil-free

2 cloves of garlic

2 tbsp of vegetable oil, for frying

3 tbsp of extra virgin olive oil

Preparation:

First, wash and cut the asparagus into 2 inch long strips.

Heat up 2 tablespoons of vegetable oil over a medium-high temperature. Add asparagus and stir-fry for several minutes. Remove from the heat and use some kitchen paper to soak the excess oil. Transfer to a serving platter and top with tuna.

Season with olive oil. Decorate with some black olives, but this is optional.

Nutritional information per serving: Kcal: 157, Protein: 17.2g, Carbs: 12.8g, Fats: 9.7g

23.   Avocado and Vegetable Soup

Ingredients:

½ large, ripe avocado

1 tbsp lemon juice

1 tbsp vegetable oil

2 small tomatoes, skinned and deseeded

1 garlic clove, crushed

1 leek, chopped

½ red chili, chopped

4 fl oz vegetable broth, unsalted

2 fl oz milk (can be replaced with almond milk for some extra taste)

Preparation:

Peel the avocado and mash the flesh with a fork. Stir in the lemon juice and set aside.

Heat the oil in a deep pot. Add the tomatoes, garlic, leek, chili and saute over a low heat for 2-3 minutes, or until softened.

Put half of the vegetable mixture in a food processor, add the mashed avocado and process until smooth. Transfer the contents to a pot.

Now add the vegetable broth and the remaining vegetables. Cover and cook for 15 minutes over a medium-low temperature.

Serve warm.

Nutritional information per serving: Kcal: 92, Protein: 2.7g, Carbs: 9.5g, Fats: 14.2g

24.   Apple Pie

Ingredients:

2 pounds of apples (I used Zestar apples, but you can really use any kind of apples you have on hand)

¼ cup of granulated sugar

¼ cup of breadcrumbs

2 tsp of cinnamon, ground

3 tbsp of freshly squeezed lemon juice

1 tsp of vanilla sugar

¼ cup of oil

1 egg, beaten

¼ cup of all-purpose flour

2 tbsp of flax seed

Pie dough

Preparation:

Preheat the oven to 375°F.

First, peel the apples and cut into bite- sized pieces. Transfer to a large bowl. I like to add about two to three tablespoons of freshly squeezed lemon juice. It gives my pie a nice sour flavor and it prevents the apples to change the color before baking. Now add breadcrumbs, vanilla sugar, granulated sugar, and cinnamon. You can also add one teaspoon of ground nutmeg in the mixture. I personally avoid it because I like the classic cinnamon taste. But you can experiment a bit. Mix well the ingredients and set aside.

On a lightly floured surface roll out the pie dough making 2 circle-shaped crusts. Grease the baking dish with some oil (or even melted butter) and place one pie crust in it. Spoon the apple mixture and cover with the remaining crust. Seal by crimping edges and brush with beaten egg.

I like to sprinkle my pie with flax seed. It adds some great nutritional values to it, but it also gives a bit of crunchy flavor I absolutely adore. This, however, is optional. You can sprinkle your pie with some nice powdered sugar instead. That really depends on your taste.

Bake for about an hour or until crust is brown and crispy. Cool for a while on a wire rack and serve.

Nutritional information per serving: Kcal: 410, Protein: 3.5g, Carbs: 56.4g, Fats: 18.8g

25.   Strawberry Coconut Salad

Ingredients:

1 cup of strawberries, halved

1 cup of apricots, sliced (fresh or canned)

1 medium-sized kiwi, peeled and sliced

1 tsp of vanilla sugar

2 tbsp of coconut flour

1 tbsp of fresh mint, finely chopped

Preparation:

Combine strawberries, apricots, and kiwi in a large bowl. Stir well and set aside.

Heat up a frying skillet over a low temperature and add coconut flour. Stir-fry constantly for about 2-3 minutes. Remove from the heat, add mint and stir well.

Pour coconut flour and mint mixture over the fruits and give it a final stir.

Refrigerate for 1 hour before serving.

Serve salad with whipped cream or cocoa powder, but this is optional.

Enjoy!

Nutritional information per serving: Kcal: 172, Protein: 4.2g, Carbs: 28.7g, Fats: 0.8g

26.   Sweet Potato with Onions

Ingredients:

4 medium sweet potatoes, peeled

6 free range eggs

2 medium-sized onions, peeled

½ tsp of turmeric

2 tsp avocado oil

Preparation:

Preheat your oven to 350 degrees. Spread some baking paper over a medium sized baking sheet. Place the potatoes on a baking sheet. Bake for about 20 minutes. Remove from the oven and allow it to cool for a while. Lower the oven heat to 200 degrees.

Meanwhile, chop the onions into small pieces. Separate egg whites from yolks. Cut the potatoes into thick slices and place them in a bowl. Add chopped onions, 2 tbsp of avocado oil, egg whites, and turmeric. Mix well.

Spread this mixture on a baking sheet and bake for another 15-20 minutes.

Nutritional information per serving: Kcal: 162, Protein: 2.2g, Carbs: 33.1g, Fats: 0.5g

27. Warm Lemon Soup

Ingredients:

1lb button mushrooms (can be replaced with shitake mushrooms)

3 tbsp of olive oil

2 cups of vegetable broth, unsalted

¼ cup of freshly squeezed lemon juice

¼ tsp of black pepper, ground

1 tsp of dried rosemary, minced

Preparation:

Heat up some oil in a deep pot. Add mushrooms and stir-fry for 3-4 minutes. Now add, vegetable broth, pepper, and rosemary. Bring it to a boil and reduce the heat to minimum. Cook for 10-12 minutes, stirring constantly.

Remove from the heat and stir in lemon juice before serving.

Nutritional information per serving: Kcal: 96, Protein: 6.3g, Carbs: 14.6g, Fats: 4.2g

28.   Nutmeg Omelet

Ingredients:

3 large eggs

1 medium onion

1 tsp of nutmeg

½ tbsp of fresh parsley, chopped

¼ tsp of black pepper, ground

Preparation:

Peel and slice the onion. Wash under the cool water and drain. Set aside. Heat up a nonstick skillet over a medium heat. In a small bowl, whisk together eggs, pepper, and parsley.

Pour the eggs in a skillet and fry for about 3 minutes. Using a spatula, remove the eggs from the frying pan and add onions and nutmeg. Stir well and return the eggs to the skillet. Cook for few more minutes, until the onions get nice golden color.

Nutritional information per serving: Kcal: 181, Protein: 10.6g, Carbs: 8.3g, Fats: 14.2g

29.   Artichoke Salad

Ingredients:

2 small pieces of turkey breast, boneless and skinless

2 large eggs

1 cup of red cabbage, grated

2 cherry tomatoes, whole

½ cup of green olives, whole

1 cup of scallions, chopped

¼ cup of artichokes, whole

2 tbsp of olive oil

2 tbsp of vegetable oil

1 tbsp of fresh lemon juice

Preparation:

Wash and pat dry the meat with a kitchen paper. Cut into 1 inch thick strips. In a large skillet, heat up the vegetable oil over a medium-high temperature. Fry the turkey strips for about 10 minutes. Remove from the heat and soak the excess oil with a kitchen paper. Transfer to a large bowl.

Meanwhile, boil the eggs. Gently place two eggs in a pot of boiling water. Cook for 10 minutes. Rinse and drain. Cool for a while and peel. You can add one teaspoon of baking soda in a boiling water. This will make the peeling process much easier. Cut the eggs into bite-sized pieces and transfer to a bowl.

Add the remaining ingredients into the bowl and mix well.

Season with fresh lemon juice.

Serve immediately.

Nutritional information per serving: Kcal: 246, Protein: 34.8g, Carbs: 19.4g, Fats: 30.2g

30.   Avocado Salsa

Ingredients:

2 ripe avocados, pitted and diced

½ cup of minced onions

2 bell peppers, seeded and minced

3 organic limes, juiced

2 tbsp of avocado oil

2 tbsp of minced fresh cilantro leaves

½ tsp of black pepper, crushed

Preparation:

Combine together all salsa ingredients in a large bowl and mix well with an electric mixer. Cover and chill until needed.

Nutritional information per serving: Kcal: 96, Protein: 1.9g, Carbs: 7.5g, Fats: 7.4g

31.   Cold Zucchini Soup

Ingredients:

1lb zucchini, trimmed and cut into chunks

2 cups of homemade chicken broth

1 small onion, peeled and finely chopped

2 garlic cloves, crushed

½ tsp of dried oregano

¼ tsp of pepper, ground

3 tbsp of vegetable oil

1 tbsp of whipping cream (optional and can be replaced with almond cream)

Preparation:

Heat oil in a large saucepan, over medium-high heat. Add chopped onion, garlic, and saute until translucent. Now add zucchini, oregano, and pepper. Continue to cook until tender.

Stir in chicken broth and bring it to a boil. Reduce the heat to minimum and cook for ten minutes.

Cool for a while and transfer to a blender. Blend until

smooth.

Stir in one tablespoon of whipping cream before serving, but this is optional.

Nutrition information per serving: Kcal: 154, Protein: 3g, Carbs: 5g, Fats: 13g

32.   Green Broccoli Risotto

Ingredients:

½ cup of rice

2 cups of fresh button mushrooms

½ cup of cooked broccoli

1 tbsp of dry rosemary

1 tsp of lime juice

½ tsp of cumin

Preparation:

First, you need to cook the rice. Wash and rinse it and put in a saucepan with 1 cup of water. Stir well and bring to the boiling point. Cover the pan with a lid and cook for about 15 minutes at a low temperature. Remove from the heat and allow it to cool.

Now you want to prepare the mushrooms. Wash and cut into similar size pieces. Heat up the grill pan over a medium temperature. Add mushrooms and stir well. Cook until all the mushrooms soften, or until all the water evaporates. Remove from the frying pan. Add cumin and mix with rice and broccoli.

Season with dry rosemary, pepper and lime juice. Serve warm.

Nutritional information per serving: Kcal: 348, Protein: 11.3g, Carbs: 55.7g, Fats: 9.6g

33.   Spinach Pie with Unsalted Goat's Cheese

Ingredients:

9 oz of fresh spinach, chopped

4 whole eggs

½ cup of goat's milk

1 cup of unsalted goat's cheese, chopped

Preparation:

Preheat an oven to a temperature of 350°F. Place a baking paper over a baking dish and set aside.

Whisk the eggs thoroughly in a mixing bowl, mix in the goat's milk and goat's cheese and whisk until well incorporated. Set aside.

Place the chopped spinach in the greased baking dish. Pour in the egg mixture and cover the spinach completely. Bake for about 40 to 45 minutes or until the cheese has melted and lightly browned.

Remove from the oven and let it rest for 5 minutes before serving.

Nutritional information per serving: Kcal: 182, Protein: 9.4g, Carbs: 14.1g, Fats: 4.2g

34.   Spring Basil Salad

Ingredients:

1 medium-sized red bell pepper, chopped in cubes

1 oz of artichokes, chopped

2 oz of pear cherry tomatoes, halved

1 small red onion, sliced

1 oz of black olives

1 tsp of basil, minced

2 oz of raw unsalted cottage cheese, crumbled

3 oz of kale, chopped and pre-cooked

½ cup of lemon juice

2 tbsp of olive oil

2 garlic cloves, crushed

½ tsp of cumin, ground

Preparation:

Combine the olive oil, lemon juice, and garlic in a small bowl. Crush the garlic and stir well to combine.

Take one large bowl and combine the veggies and cheese. Drizzle with some marinade and serve immediately.

Nutritional information per serving: Kcal: 353, Protein: 7.9g, Carbs: 23.8g, Fats: 28.2g

35.   Roasted Veggies

Ingredients:

½ cup of beetroot, peeled and diced

½ cup of green beans, cooked and drained

½ cup of brussel sprouts, chopped

½ cup of pumpkin, peeled and chopped

½ cup of carrot, chopped

1 cup of fresh tomatoes, roughly chopped

½ cup of roasted tomatoes

1 small onion, sliced

½ cup of cooked lentils

1 cup of finely chopped silverbeet

1 cup of raw goat's cheese, unsalted

Preparation:

Preheat the oven to 350 degrees. In a large bowl, combine beetroot, green beans, brussel sprouts and pumpkin. Place on an oven tray and bake for about 20 minutes.

Meanwhile, heat up a medium sized, non-stick saucepan.

Add onions and carrot and fry for about 5 minutes, stirring constantly.

Add diced tomatoes and silverbeet. Gently simmer for about 20 minutes. Add silverbeet and salt. Serve the lentils topped with roasted vegetables, roasted tomatoes and goat's cheese.

Nutritional information per serving: Kcal: 102, Protein: 7.4g, Carbs: 13.4g, Fats: 6.1g

36.   Brussel Sprouts Soup with Lemon

Ingredients:

8oz fresh brussel sprouts

A handful of fresh parsley, finely chopped

1 tsp of dry thyme

1 tbsp of fresh lemon juice

Preparation:

Place the brussel sprouts in a deep pot and pour enough water to cover. Bring it to a boil and cook until tender. Remove from the heat and drain.

Transfer to a food processor. Add fresh parsley, thyme, and about ½ cup of water. Pulse until smooth mixture. Return to a pot and add some more water. Bring it to a boil and cook for several minutes, over a minimum temperature. Season with fresh lemon juice. Serve warm.

Nutritional information per serving: Kcal: 87, Protein: 3.5g, Carbs: 7.6g, Fats: 5.3g

37.   Warm Quinoa with Plums

Ingredients:

1 cup of quinoa

1 cup of plums, cut in half and pitted

1 tbsp of brown sugar

½ tsp of cinnamon, ground

Water

Preparation:

Put your plums in a large skillet and add enough water to cover. Bring it to boil and cook for 10 minutes, or until tender. Remove from the heat and drain. Set aside.

Use the same skillet to boil 2 cups of water. Add quinoa, sugar, and cinnamon. Reduce the heat to minimum and cook until slightly thickened. This should take about 5 minutes. Remove from the heat and pour into bowls. Top with plums.

Nutritional information per serving: Kcal: 150, Protein: 7.7g, Carbs: 5.8g, Fats: 0.2g

38.   Swedish Salad

Ingredients:

4 oz of cottage cheese, crumbled

6 oz of smoked salmon, cut into strips

½ cup of fresh basil, finely chopped

1 cup of Iceberg lettuce, finely chopped

¼ cup of lamb's lettuce, chopped

1 cup of radicchio, finely chopped

For dressing:

2 tbsp of wine vinegar

2 tbsp of olive oil

1 tsp of black pepper, ground

1 tbsp of brown sugar

1 tsp of dill, ground

Preparation:

Preheat the frying skillet over a medium-high temperature. Add sugar and stir constantly until caramelized. Add the vinegar and cook for about 1 minute more. Remove from the heat and let cool for a while. Add dill, stir, and set aside.

Combine basil, lettuce, lamb's lettuce and radicchio on a serving plate. In another bowl, combine cheese, salmon and olive oil. Pour it over the salad.

Spoon the dressing over the salad and season with a pinch of pepper to taste.

Serve immediately!

Nutritional information per serving: Kcal: 227, Protein: 13.8g, Carbs: 9.8g, Fats: 17.6g

39.   Button Mushroom Soup with Carrots

Ingredients:

1 medium-sized carrot, diced

½ cup of shredded coconut

1 cup of coconut milk

1 cup of button mushrooms, thinly sliced

5 cups of water

1 tsp of white pepper, ground

1 celery, finely chopped

1 tbsp of olive oil

1 green chili, chopped, seed removed

3 onions, chopped

A handful of fresh parsley, finely chopped

Preparation:

Heat the olive oil in a deep pot. Throw in the onions, carrots, and shredded coconut. Toss for about 5 minutes and then add the mushroom to it. Stir-fry for another 5 minutes.

Now add the celery and the chili to the pot. Season to taste and pour the milk and water. Reduce the heat, cover, and cook for 20 minutes.

Remove from the heat and sprinkle with parsley.

Serve warm.

Nutrition information per serving: Kcal: 130, Protein: 2.3g, Carbs: 9.2g, Fats: 14.4g

40.   Eggplant French Toast

Ingredients:

1 large eggplant

3 free range eggs

¼ tsp of sea salt

1 tbsp of vegetable oil

½ tsp of cinnamon

Preparation:

Peel eggplant and cut lengthwise into slices. Sprinkle salt on each side of eggplant. Allow it to rest for few minutes. Rinse well and press gently to drain and extract any excess liquid.

Meanwhile, mix eggs with cinnamon in a large bowl. Heat up a non-stick frying pan over a medium temperature.

Put your eggplant slices in egg mixture. Make few holes with a knife to allow the mixture to permeate the eggplant. Fry it until golden brown color, on each side. Serve your 'French toast' warm.

Nutritional information per serving: Kcal: 78, Protein: 5.5g, Carbs: 9.8g, Fats: 6.3g

41.   Flan Steak Salad

Ingredients:

For the meat:

8oz flan steak

1 tbsp of dried oregano, chopped

3 tbsp of dijon mustard

3 tbsp of olive oil

¼ tsp of pepper

For salad:

3.5oz red radish, sliced

1 large onion, peeled and sliced

A handful of arugula, torn

A handful of lettuce, torn

For dressing:

¼ cup of olive oil

1 tbsp of apple cider vinegar

½ tsp of chili pepper, ground

Preparation:

Combine dressing ingredients in a small bowl. Stir well and set aside.

Preheat the grill pan over medium-high heat. Wash and pat dry steaks. Slice into 1 inch thick slices. Set aside.

Combine olive oil with mustard, pepper, and oregano. Using a kitchen brush, spread this mixture over each meat slice and grill for about 10-12 minutes, stirring regularly. When the meat has lightly browned and charred, remove from the heat and place in a bowl.

Add sliced onion, lettuce, radish, and arugula. Toss well to combine. I like to sprinkle some cayenne pepper over onions before I mix them with other vegetables. This, however, is optional.

Now combine all dressing ingredients in a small bowl. Drizzle over salad and serve immediately.

Nutritional information per serving: Kcal: 450, Protein: 41g, Carbs: 10.2g, Fats: 27.8g

42.   Rice Pudding with Almond Milk

Ingredients:

½ cup of uncooked rice

2 cups of almond milk

½ cup of cranberries

Preparation:

Use package instructions to cook the rice.

Pour 2 cups of milk in a medium-sized pan and bring it to a boil. Stir in cooked rice. Cook for 20 minutes more, until you get a creamy mixture.

Stir in cranberries and remove from the heat. Allow it to cool in the refrigerator before serving.

Nutritional information per serving: Kcal: 282, Protein: 5.3g, Carbs: 57.5g, Fats: 3.9g

43. Mushroom Omelet

Ingredients:

1 cup of button mushrooms, sliced

2 large eggs

1 tsp of fresh rosemary, chopped

¼ tsp of dry oregano

Preparation:

Heat up a large non-stick skillet, over a medium temperature. Add button mushrooms and cook for 3-4 minutes, until the water evaporates. Remove from the skillet.

In a small bowl, whisk together eggs, rosemary, and oregano. Pour the mixture into the skillet and fry for about 4 minutes. When eggs are set, layer half of the skillet with mushrooms. Fold untopped half of the omelet over filling and fry for one more minute. Move to a plate and serve with few lettuce leaves, but this is optional.

Nutritional information per serving: Kcal: 98, Protein: 6.3g, Carbs: 2.4g, Fats: 6.7g

44.   Sweet Potatoes with Brussel Sprouts

Ingredients:

1 lb of Brussel sprouts

5 medium-sized sweet potatoes, chopped

2 red onions, peeled and sliced

¼ cup of lime juice

1 tbsp of fresh parsley, finely chopped

3 tbsp of olive oil

Preparation:

Preheat oven to 300°F.

Heat up the oil in a large skillet. Heat up over a medium temperature and add onion slices. Cook until translucent, 4-5 minutes.

Meanwhile, peel and cut potatoes into bite size cubes and cut Brussel sprouts in half. Add potatoes and Brussel sprouts in a frying pan and reduce the heat to minimum. Stir well until nicely coated and simmer for about 10 minutes. Remove from the heat.

Transfer the vegetables to a baking sheet. Season with

parsley. Roast for about 30-40 minutes, or until tender. Remove from the oven and allow it to cool for a while.

Sprinkle with fresh lime juice before serving.

Nutritional information per serving: Kcal: 186, Protein: 5.5g, Carbs: 36.2g, Fats: 5.5g

45. Coconut Sugar Puree

Ingredients:

2 large apples, peeled and cored

2 tbsp of pumpkin seeds

3 tbsp of coconut palm sugar

1 tbsp of flax seeds, whole

1 tbsp of flaxseed oil, cold-pressed

1 tsp of cinnamon

Preparation:

Roughly chop the apples and place them in a pot. Add enough water to cover and cook until soft. This should take about 20 minutes.

Remove from the heat and drain. Allow the apples to cool for a while and transfer to a food processor. Add other ingredients and pulse until incorporated.

Chill for a while before serving.

Nutritional information per serving: Kcal: 250, Protein: 0.8g, Carbs: 19.5g, Fats: 1.7g

46.   Cold Apple Dessert

Ingredients:

4 medium-sized apples

½ cup of almonds, minced

½ cup of walnuts, minced

1 tsp of cinnamon

1 tsp of stevia

2 tbsp of coconut oil

Preparation:

Peel and slice the apples. Transfer to a deep pot and add enough water to cover. Cook the apples until soft. Remove from the pot and drain.

Combine the ingredients with an electric mixer or a food processor. Place the mixture onto the parchment paper and dehydrate at 115 degrees F for 7-9 hours. The mixture is completely dehydrated when the paper peels off easily.

Slice into 3x3 inches pieces and serve cold.

Nutritional information per serving: Kcal: 228, Protein: 2.5g, Carbs: 42.2g, Fats: 5.1g

47.   Orange Ice Cream

Ingredients:

1 cup of raw coconut cream

¼ cup of macadamia nuts, minced

¼ cup of fresh orange juice

2-3 drops of natural orange essential oil

1 tsp of orange zest

3 tsp of stevia

1 tbsp of coconut oil

Preparation:

Combine the ingredients in a large bowl. Use an electric mixer to get a smooth mixture. Pour the mixture into ice cream containers and freeze overnight.

Nutritional information per serving: Kcal: 162, Protein: 2.8g, Carbs: 18.7g, Fats: 10.3g

48.   Orange Sutlac

Ingredients:

1 cup of cooked rice

2 cups of almond milk

½ cup of fresh orange juice

1 tsp of stevia

½ tsp of cinnamon

Preparation:

Follow the package instructions to cook rice. Reduce the heat to minimum and add almond milk and stevia. Stir well for about 15 minutes.

Remove from the heat and add orange juice. Pour it into small bowls. Allow it to cool well in the refrigerator before serving.

Sprinkle some cinnamon on top, but this is optional.

Nutritional information per serving: Kcal: 169, Protein: 5.6g, Carbs: 32.5g, Fats: 3.8g

49.   Lemon Carrot Sticks

Ingredients:

5 medium-sized carrots

1 organic lemon, sliced into wedges

1 tbsp of fresh rosemary, chopped

For the Marinade:

1 tsp of minced garlic

1 cup of organic lemon juice

½ tsp of dried thyme leaves

½ tsp of dried oregano

Preparation:

Combine together all marinade ingredients in a medium bowl. Mix until well combined.

Place the carrots and coat evenly with the marinade mixture. Cover the bowl and chill for at least 1 hour to marinate.

Preheat the grill to high heat. Place the carrots and add ½ cup of lemon marinade. Grill for about 15 minutes, stirring constantly. Add some more marinade if necessary. Transfer to a serving platter.

Serve warm with lemons wedges and sprinkle with minced parsley.

Nutritional information per serving: Kcal: 92, Protein: 1.4g, Carbs: 4.8g, Fats: 0.9g

50.   Smoked Paprika Mushrooms

Ingredients:

¼ cup of chopped fresh coriander leaves

3 garlic cloves, minced

¼ cup of lemon juice

1 cup of button mushrooms

½ teaspoon smoked paprika

½ teaspoon cumin, ground

½ teaspoon dry parsley

Preparation:

Add the coriander, garlic, paprika, cumin, parsley and lemon juice in a food processor and pulse to combine. Gradually add in the oil and mix the ingredients until a smooth mixture.

Transfer the mixture into a bowl, add the mushrooms and gently toss to coat the mushrooms evenly with sauce. Chill for at least 2 hours to allow the flavors to penetrate into the mushrooms.

Remove the mushrooms from the chiller and preheat the

grill pan. Place the mushrooms and grill for about 3 to 4 minutes on each side. Add some marinade while cooking.

Remove the mushrooms from the grill, transfer to a serving plate and serve with lemon wedges or some vegetables.

Nutritional information per serving: Kcal: 301, Protein: 8.4g, Carbs: 55.7g, Fats: 0.6g

51. English Muffins

Ingredients:

1 cup of all-purpose flour

¼ cup of brown sugar

1 tsp of yeast

1 tbsp of butter, melted

2 cups of skim milk

Preparation:

Combine dry ingredients in a large bowl and mix well. Now gently stir in 1 tablespoon of melted butter and milk, until the dough forms a ball. You can add some more milk to get the right consistency. Mix well for few minutes, using your hands or an electric mixer. The dough will become very sticky.

Now add some more flour (2 tablespoons should be enough) to get a nice and smooth mixture. Cover and let it rise for about 15 minutes.

Meanwhile, preheat the oven to 350°F. Use a muffin molds to shape your muffins. Bake for about 20 minutes, until nice gold brown color. Remove from the oven and serve.

Nutritional information per serving: Kcal: 141, Protein: 5.2g, Carbs: 27.3g, Fats: 1.2g

52.   Pumpkin Pancakes

Ingredients:

5 egg whites

½ tablespoon cinnamon

¼ cup oats

½ tbsp of sugar

1 tbsp of flax, ground

1/3 cup of fresh pumpkin, canned or mashed

Preparation:

Combine all ingredients in a large bowl and mix well.

Now, heat up the frying pan over a medium temperature until it's fully hot. Keep the constant temperature throughout the whole baking process.

Use a big spoon to put the blended ingredients on the frying pan.

This is the easiest part. You simply have to make pancakes now the usual way.

Nutritional information per serving: Kcal: 164, Protein: 4.2g, Carbs: 27.5g, Fats: 0.5g

53.   Creamy Parsley Salad

Ingredients:

1 large cucumber, sliced

1 large tomato, roughly chopped

3 spring onions, chopped

A handful of parsley, chopped

¼ cup of ricotta, unsalted

3 tbsp of vegetable oil

1 tbsp of coconut oil

3 tbsp of freshly squeezed lime juice

Preparation:

Combine the vegetable oil with coconut oil and lime juice. Stir well.

Now place the vegetables in a large bowl and stir to combine. Drizzle with some marinade and serve.

You can add some ricotta, but this is optional.

Nutritional information per serving: Kcal: 105, Protein: 3.2g, Carbs: 14.7g, Fats: 5.3g

54.   Chocolate Chip Cookies

Ingredients:

2 large eggs

2 cups of chocolate chips

1 cup of unsalted butter

1 pinch of ground cinnamon

2 ½ cups of all-purpose flour

½ teaspoon baking soda

2 ½ cups brown sugar

Preparation:

Preheat your oven to 370°F. Take a bowl and toss in the butter and brown sugar. Mix together until they form a fluffy mixture. Then, add the eggs and mix till it combines with the other ingredients.

Take a separate bowl and put in the baking soda, flour and cinnamon. Mix the ingredients together.

Add the contents of the second bowl to the first bowl. Use your hands to stir in the chocolate chips into the mixture. Put the mixture onto the baking sheet and add a pinch of salt on to each cookie. Bake the cookies till they are golden brown, which should take around 10 minutes.

Nutritional information per serving: Kcal: 49, Protein: 0.6g, Carbs: 6.2g, Fats: 2.8g

55.   Blueberry Yogurt

Ingredients:

½ cup of blueberries

½ cup of orange juice

1 ½ cups of plain yogurt

1 cup of strawberries

1 banana, sliced

1 tbsp of honey

Preparation:

Put all the ingredients in food processor. Blend for about one minute or until smooth. If necessary, add more orange juice.

Transfer the mixture to the serving glass. Refrigerate 30 minutes before using.

Nutritional information per serving: Kcal: 189, Protein: 6.8g, Carbs: 41.5g, Fats: 1.2g

56.   Grilled Chicken Breast Salad

Ingredients:

1 large chicken breast, boneless and skinless, cut into bite-sized pieces

1 large tomato, chopped

1 medium-sized green pepper, finely chopped

1 large cucumber, sliced

A handful of fresh lettuce, torn

1 medium-sized red bell pepper, finely chopped

A handful of fresh parsley, chopped

4 tbsp of olive oil

For dressing:

¼ cup of fresh lime juice

3 tbsp of olive oil

½ small shallot, minced

1 garlic clove, crushed

Preparation:

Heat up the olive oil over a medium-high heat. Add chicken breast and stir-fry for 5-7 minutes, stirring constantly. Remove from the heat and set aside.

Place vegetables in a large bowl, add chicken breast, and toss to combine.

In a small bowl, combine dressing ingredients and whisk well with a spoon. Drizzle over salad and serve.

Nutritional information per serving: Kcal: 171, Protein: 31g, Carbs: 15.5g, Fats: 25g

57.   Apple Muesli with Goji Berries

Ingredients:

1 cup rolled oats

½ cup dried goji berries

2 large apples

3 tbsp of flaxseeds

3 tbsp of honey

1 ¼ cups of coconut water

1 ¼ cups of plain yogurt

2 tbsp mint leaves

Preparation:

Grate the apples into a large bowl.

Put the yogurt, Goji berries, flax seeds, rolled oats, mint and coconut water in the bowl and mix well. Leave the mixture in the fridge overnight.

Spoon the honey into the muesli and serve!

Nutritional information per serving: Kcal: 420, Protein: 13.2g, Carbs: 57.4g, Fats: 6.1g

58.   Breakfast Burrito

Ingredients:

2 slices of organic deli meat

1 tbsp of butter

2 whole eggs

¼ cup of chopped spinach

2 tbsp of bell pepper, finely chopped

1 small tomato, chopped

1 tsp of fresh cilantro,

Preparation:

Whisk the eggs and cilantro in a mixing bowl and set aside.

In a pan, apply medium-high heat and add the butter. Sauté the spinach, tomato and bell pepper for 3 minutes. Add the eggs and scramble the mixture with a spatula. When the scrambled egg is done, remove from heat and add into each sliced deli meat.

Roll the ham and secure the end with a tooth pick. Brown the deli meat evenly on all sides and transfer to a serving plate. Serve warm.

Nutritional information per serving: Kcal: 395, Protein: 21.6g, Carbs: 19.4g, Fats: 17.1g

59.   Creamy Asparagus Soup

Ingredients:

6oz of fresh asparagus, chopped, woody ends discarded

3 spring onions, finely chopped

2 garlic cloves, crushed

2 tbsp of freshly squeezed lime juice

2 cups of vegetable broth, unsalted

½ cup of whipping cream

¼ tsp of black pepper, ground

1 bay leaf

Preparation:

Heat the oil over a medium temperature in a deep pan. Fry the asparagus for 2-3 minutes to soften. Add the onions, garlic, and pepper. Stir-fry for another two minutes.

Now add the vegetable broth and bay leaf. Bring it to a boil. Cook for five minutes and remove from the heat.

Transfer to a blender. Add sour cream and pulse to combine.

Stir in lime juice and serve.

Nutritional information per serving: Kcal: 115, Protein: 19g, Carbs: 15.7g, Fats: 4.6

60.   Veggie Wraps

Ingredients:

1 cup of cherry tomatoes, cut in half

1 cup of red cabbage, finely chopped

½ cup of green beans, cooked

1 tsp of dry parsley

2 tbsp of fresh lemon juice

1 tbsp of brown sugar

1 tsp of dry oregano

4 very large romaine lettuce leaves

½ tsp of red pepper, ground

Preparation:

In a large skillet, combine the tomatoes, oregano and red pepper. Stir well and fry for 2-3 minutes, over a medium temperature. Season with pepper. Now you can add the remaining ingredients and cover. Let it stand for about 10 minutes.

Divide the mixture up among the leaves and wrap. Secure wraps with toothpicks.

Serve.

Nutritional information per serving: Kcal: 400, Protein: 9.2g, Carbs: 61.3g, Fats: 18.6g

61.   Chicken Soup with Garlic

Ingredients:

5 oz of chicken breast, boneless and skinless

1 tbsp of parsley, freshly grounded

5 garlic cloves, finely chopped

1 small onion, chopped

1 tbsp of almond flour

4 tbsp of vegetable oil

¼ tsp of black pepper, ground

Preparation:

Preheat 2 tablespoons of vegetable oil in a frying skillet over a medium-high temperature. Add onion and 3 garlic cloves. Stir-fry until translucent.

Transfer onion and garlic in a deep pot. Add meat, parsley, and season with pepper. Pour enough water to cover all ingredients. Reduce the heat, cover and cook for 30 minutes.

Drain the soup in a large bowl. Chop the meat into bite-size pieces.

Heat up 2 tablespoons of oil in a deep pot over a medium-high temperature. Transfer the meat again into the pot with 2 garlic cloves and fry for 1 minute. Add the flour and stir constantly for 2-3 minutes.

Finally, pour the soup into the pot and give it a final stir. Cook for about 10 minutes more. Stir occasionally.

Serve warm.

Nutritional information per serving: Kcal: 93, Protein: 12.8g, Carbs: 16.5g, Fats: 22.4g

62.   Banana Nut Porridge

Ingredients:

1 ripe yellow banana, sliced

2 cups of unsweetened coconut milk

½ tablespoon of cinnamon

½ cup chopped cashews

½ cup chopped almonds

½ cup chopped pecans

Preparation:

In a mixing bowl, place the nuts and pour in with just enough water to cover. Cover the bowl and soak overnight. Drain and rinse with running water. Transfer into a food processor together with the banana, coconut milk and cinnamon. Process the ingredients until thick and smooth.

Place the mixture in a pan over medium-high heat. Cook for about 5 minutes, or until it reaches to a boil while stirring regularly. Portion into 4 individual serving bowls and serve with extra chopped nuts if desired.

Nutritional information per serving: Kcal: 306, Protein: 7.3g, Carbs: 17.6g, Fats: 25.6g

63.   Cheesy Spinach and Tomato Omelet

Ingredients:

4 medium free-range whole eggs, beaten

½ cup of raw cottage cheese, unsalted

½ cup of white onion, diced

1 cup of fresh spinach, finely chopped

6 pieces of cherry tomatoes, diced

1 tbsp of butter

¼ tsp of black pepper, ground

Preparation:

Add the butter in a skillet and apply with medium heat. When the butter has melted, sauté the onions until soft and pour in the beaten eggs. Cook for about 3 minutes or until the bottom part is lightly brown.

Add the cheese, spinach and tomatoes on one side of the egg and season to taste with pepper. Carefully lift the other side of the omelet and flip it over to cover the vegetables. Reduce the heat to low and cook for about 2 minutes.

Slide the omelet onto a serving plate and serve with extra

cheese on top.

Nutritional information per serving: Kcal: 210, Protein: 18.3g, Carbs: 4.6g, Fats: 14.8g

64.   Hawaii Salad

Ingredients:

½ of small watermelon, peeled and cubed

1 large ripe avocado, peeled, pit removed, and sliced into bite-sized pieces

1 tbsp of fresh ginger, shredded

1 tsp of fresh mint, finely chopped

1 cup of lemon juice

Preparation:

Combine all dry ingredients in a large serving bowl. Pour over the lemon juice and stir well. Refrigerate for about 30 minutes before serving.

Nutritional information per serving: Kcal: 149, Protein: 1.6g, Carbs: 22.7g, Fats: 0.4g

65.   Almond Meal Pancakes

Ingredients:

1 cup of almond flour

2 medium free-range whole eggs

½ cup of water

½ tsp of baking soda

¼ tsp of sugar

2 tbsp of ghee

Preparation:

Combine flour and baking soda in a mixing bowl and set aside.

In a separate bowl, whisk together the eggs, sugar and 1 tablespoon of ghee until well combined. Pour the egg mixture into the bowl with the flour mixture and mix it thoroughly until smooth. If the batter mixture is too thick, add water and mix until the desired consistency is achieved. Cover the bowl with a cloth and let it sit for 15 minutes, set aside.

Add the remaining ghee into a pan and apply with medium-high heat. Once the ghee is hot, pour in enough pancake mixture just to cover the base of the pan. Cook until the bottom part is lightly browned and flip it over to cook the other side. Repeat the procedure with the remaining pancake mixture and place them on a serving platter.

Serve warm with your favorite spread, if desired.

Nutritional information per serving: Kcal: 150, Protein: 6.2g, Carbs: 4.3g, Fats: 13.6g

66.   Beets Ricotta Salad

Ingredients:

5 oz of beets, peeled and cut into wedges

2 large oranges, peeled and chopped

1 cup of arugula, chopped

½ cup of unsalted Ricotta cheese, crumbled

¼ tsp of black pepper

1 tsp of chia seeds

2 tbsp of extra virgin olive oil

Preparation:

Place the beets in a large skillet over a medium-high temperature. Cook for 10 minutes, or until soften. Remove from the heat and drain. Set aside.

Meanwhile, combine oil, pepper and chia seeds in a mixing bowl. Stir well and set aside.

Combine arugula, oranges, and beets on a serving plate. Top with ricotta cheese and season with previously prepared dressing.

Serve.

Nutritional information per serving: Kcal: 134, Protein: 8.6g, Carbs: 15.3g, Fats: 10.4g

67.   Creamy Spinach Chicken Breast

Ingredients:

1 lb of chicken breast, boneless and skinless

2 cups of spinach, chopped

1 cup of yogurt, low-fat

3 green peppers

3 chili peppers

2 small onions, chopped

1 tbsp of ginger, ground

1 tsp of red pepper, ground

4 tbsp of vegetable oil

Preparation:

Wash and pat dry the chicken using a kitchen paper. Chop into bite size pieces. Finely chop onion and peppers and set aside.

Heat up the oil in a large weasel. Add onions and peppers and sauté for few minutes. Now add chicken breast pieces, and sprinkle with ground ginger and red pepper. Stir-fry for ten minutes, or until the chicken turns light brown.

Meanwhile, combine low fat yogurt with spinach in a food processor. Mix well for 30 seconds. Add this mixture to the weasel and fry until the spinach gets well mashed.

Cover the weasel, remove from the heat and let it stand for about 10 minutes before serving.

Nutritional information per serving: Kcal: 292, Protein: 26.4g, Carbs: 7.2g, Fats: 18.3g

68.   Pirate Salad

Ingredients:

2 medium-sized apples, peeled and cut into bite-sized pieces

2 large oranges, peeled and cut into wedges

2 large bananas, peeled and sliced

2 kiwi, peeled and sliced

1 tbsp of rum

1 cup of lemon juice

1 tbsp of sugar

1 tsp of lemon zest

Preparation:

Combine apples, oranges and bananas in a large bowl. Pour over ½ cup of lemon juice and stir well. Add kiwi and bananas and give it a final stir.

Combine the rest of lemon juice with rum and lemon zest in a small mixing bowl. Pour over the salad and refrigerate for 1 hour before use.

You can serve it with ice cream or add any other fruit by

your taste.

Enjoy!

Nutritional information per serving: Kcal: 142, Protein: 1.7g, Carbs: 43.5g, Fats: 0.3g

69.   Red Bean Puree Casserole

Ingredients:

1 cup of red beans, pre-cooked

½ cup of green beans

½ cup of button mushrooms

1 cup of cottage cheese, unsalted

1 cup of Greek yogurt

2 egg whites

2 tbsp of olive oil

Preparation:

Combine the ingredients in a food processor. Mix well for 30 seconds. Preheat the oven to 300°F.

Coat the small baking dish with 2 tablespoons of olive oil. Pour the red beans mixture in a baking dish and bake for about 10-15 minutes. You want to get a nice light brown color. Remove from the oven, let it stand for about 10 minutes and cut into 4 equal pieces.

Serve warm.

Nutritional information per serving: Kcal: 259, Protein: 15.7g, Carbs: 46.4g, Fats: 8.5g

70.   Greek Style Chicken

Ingredients:

4 pieces of chicken breast halves

1 cup of cottage cheese, unsalted

½ cup of Greek yogurt

1 cup of cucumber, chopped

1 cup of lettuce, chopped

1 cup of cherry tomatoes

½ cup of onions, chopped

5 garlic cloves, finely chopped

2 tbsp of fresh lemon juice

1 tbsp of dried oregano, minced

½ tsp of red pepper, ground

3 tbsp of olive oil

6 whole-wheat pitas, cut into wedges

Preparation:

Wash and cut the meat into small pieces. Set aside.

Combine the cottage cheese, Greek yogurt, vegetables and spices in a food processor. Mix well for 30 seconds.

Heat up the olive oil over a medium temperature. Fry chicken chops for about 20 minutes, stirring constantly. Add the vegetable mixture to the saucepan. Stir well and cook for another 10 minutes. Remove from the heat and shape this mixture into 6 equal parts.

Serve with pitas.

Nutritional information per serving: Kcal: 490, Protein: 46.2g, Carbs: 22.5g, Fats: 24.4g

71.   Unsalted Cottage Cheese with Veggies

Ingredients:

½ cup of cottage cheese, unsalted

1 small onion, chopped

1 small carrot, sliced

1 small tomato, sliced

2 medium-sized bell peppers

1 tbsp of olive oil

Preparation:

Wash and pat dry the vegetables using a kitchen paper. Cut into thin slices or strips.

Heat up the olive oil over a medium temperature and fry the vegetables for about 10 minutes, stirring constantly. You want to wait until the vegetables soften, then add cottage cheese. Stir well. Fry for another 2-3 minutes.

Remove from the heat and serve.

Nutritional information per serving: Kcal: 175, Protein: 15.5g, Carbs: 7.3g, Fats: 9.2g

72.   Simple Lime Salad

Ingredients:

½ medium-sized chicken breast, boneless and skinless

½ cucumber, sliced

1 small tomato, roughly chopped

1 cup of fresh lettuce, torn

1 small green pepper, sliced

1 tbsp of lime juice

3 tbsp of olive oil

Preparation:

Wash and pat dry the meat. Chop into bite-sized pieces.

Heat up the olive oil over medium-high heat. Add chopped chicken breast and fry for about 10-15 minutes, or until lightly charred. Remove from the heat and cool for a while.

Meanwhile, combine the vegetables in a glass jar. Add the meat and mix well. Season with salt lime juice. Seal the lid and you're ready to go.

Nutrition information per serving: Kcal: 70, Protein: 7.9g, Carbs: 11g, Fats: 2.4g

73.   Roasted Lentils

Ingredients:

½ cups of lentils, raw

2 tbsp of olive oil

1 tsp of black pepper, ground

1 tsp of red chili, ground

1 tsp of cinnamon, ground

Preparation:

First you want to cook lentils. Pour about 2 cups of water in a saucepan and bring it to boil. Add lentils and boil for about 15-20 minutes, until soft from inside and still hold their shape. Remove from the heat and rinse well with cold water. Drain the lentils and set aside.

Preheat the oven to 300 degrees. In a large bowl, coat the lentils with salt, olive oil, pepper, red chili powder and cinnamon. Spread the lentils over a medium sized baking dish and bake for about 20 minutes.

Prepared like this, lentils can be stored in the air-tight container for about 15 days.

Nutritional information per serving: Kcal: 238, Protein: 28g, Carbs: 19.5g, Fats: 8.5g

ADDITIONAL TITLES FROM THIS AUTHOR

70 Effective Meal Recipes to Prevent and Solve Being Overweight: Burn Fat Fast by Using Proper Dieting and Smart Nutrition

By

Joe Correa CSN

48 Acne Solving Meal Recipes: The Fast and Natural Path to Fixing Your Acne Problems in Less Than 10 Days!

By

Joe Correa CSN

41 Alzheimer's Preventing Meal Recipes: Reduce or Eliminate Your Alzheimer's Condition in 30 Days or Less!

By

Joe Correa CSN

70 Effective Breast Cancer Meal Recipes: Prevent and Fight Breast Cancer with Smart Nutrition and Powerful Foods

By

Joe Correa CSN

www.ingramcontent.com/pod-product-compliance
Lightning Source LLC
Chambersburg PA
CBHW030244030426
42336CB00009B/244